Like Cats
And Dogs

Kenneth Jernigan
Editor

Large Type Edition

#12

A KERNEL BOOK
published by
NATIONAL FEDERATION OF THE BLIND

TABLE OF CONTENTS

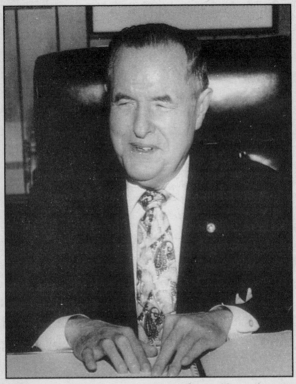

Kenneth Jernigan, President Emeritus
National Federation of the Blind

EDITOR'S INTRODUCTION

*I*n the early and mid 1930s, when I was a boy in grade school, I dearly loved to read poetry--or, more properly speaking, have poetry read to me. And my teachers often obliged. One of my favorites was a poem by Eugene Field called the "Gingham Dog and the Calico Cat." Although it will never be considered a classic, I liked it. It begins like this:

"The gingham dog and the calico cat
Side by side on the table sat;

'Twas half-past twelve, and (what do you think!)
Nor one nor t'other had slept a wink!"

The poem goes on to tell how the cat and dog had an awful fight and concludes by giving the outcome:

"But the truth about the cat and pup
Is this: they ate each other up!"

Thus, we come to the title of this book,

Like Cats and Dogs. Maybe I chose it because I once had a dog that I dearly loved, or because I currently have some adorable kittens--or maybe because of the well-known saying about people fighting like cats and dogs. Regardless of the reason, the title is chosen, and we come to a question: Exactly how do cats and dogs behave toward each other?

If they don't understand each other, they fight "like cats and dogs." But if they have the opportunity to get acquainted, they can live in harmony and become good friends.

As it is with cats and dogs, so it can be with the blind and their sighted neighbors. There can either be harmony and friendship or misunderstanding and frustration. This little volume (the twelfth in the Kernel Book series) is meant to promote understanding, the ultimate framework of all true friendship and mutual respect.

As with past Kernel Books, the stories here are real-life experiences, told by the blind persons who lived them. The one exception is the article by Theresa House, who is the sighted wife of a blind man. Her parents feared that a blind person could never be an adequate husband for their daughter, and certainly not a suitable father for her children. You will see how it is turning out as they live their lives and raise their family.

As a matter of fact, marriage and children are major themes of this book. Bruce Gardner, blind and preparing to be a lawyer, dates and falls in love with a young sighted woman. She has questions, and so do her father and mother.

And there is the matter of blind parents and sighted children. As the boy and girl grow up, how do they feel? Do they think their parents can take care of them--and how do the parents feel? What ambitions do the parents have for their children?

There is another theme relative to children (blind children). Many are not given the chance to learn Braille. What does that do to them, and how do they feel about it as they come to adulthood?

There is more--the article I wrote about the difference between the sounds and smells of today and sixty years ago, the story about a blind kitten (told by the owner, of course, not the kitten), an account of a blind woman's experience with pouring coffee, and much else. But I think I have told you enough to give you an inkling of what to expect.

At the core, all of the people represented here are talking about the same thing. What they are saying is this: In everything that counts we who are blind are just like you. As you read, you will recognize yourself in the story of our experiences. We laugh and cry, work and play, hope and dream, just like you. And although we don't forget that we are blind, we don't constantly think about it either. We are concerned with the routine business of daily living--what we plan to have for dinner, the latest gossip, and the current shenanigans in Washington.

Around fifty thousand people become blind in this country each year. That means that it may happen to you, a member of your family, a neighbor, or a friend. So we want you to know what blindness is like--and, more to the point, what it isn't like. That is why we are producing the Kernel Books. We hope you will find this volume both informative and interesting. If you do, we will have accomplished our purpose. We want to live in harmony with our neighbors--not the way most people think cats and dogs live.

Kenneth Jernigan
Baltimore, Maryland
1997

THE SMELLS AND SOUNDS OF SIXTY YEARS
by Kenneth Jernigan

*E*verybody knows that change is probably the only constant in life, but I think we don't fully understand what that means until after we're fifty. At least, that is how it has been with me.

As readers of the Kernel Books know, I grew up on a farm in rural Tennessee in the 1920s and '30s, and it seems to me that almost nothing today is the way it was then. Since I have been blind all of my life, I am not talking about how things look but how they smell, taste, sound, and feel.

Start with smell. The world smells different today from what it did then. Nowadays I spend much of my time indoors, breathing conditioned air, whether heated or cooled. But that wasn't the way it was when I was a boy.

Since we didn't have electricity, we couldn't have had air conditioning even if we had been able to afford it. So in the summer the windows were open, and usually so were the doors.

The air was rich with odors--the smell of growing things, of the barnyard, of the dust and gasoline from an occasional passing car, and of creeks. These were the smells of summer, but there were also the smells of winter--wood burning in the fireplace, the smell of the unheated portions of the house, and the smell of the country in winter.

And it was not just the odors of that time but also the sounds--the mixture of stillness, bird songs, distant cattle, and the aliveness of the land. Today, whether indoors or out, one thing is always present--the sound of motors. There are automobiles, office machines, fluorescent lights, power tools, lawn mowers, vacuum cleaners, kitchen appliances, air conditioners, and heating units.

When I was a boy on the farm, I might go a whole week without hearing a motor--but not today. In the world of the '90s, there is never a minute without a motor. Sometimes it is an avalanche of noise, and sometimes only a vibration in the background--but it is always there--always a motor.

And I mustn't omit taste and touch. At first thought, it might seem that there would be no difference between then and now, but there is. It isn't necessarily that I can't touch most of the things today that I touched in the 1930s. It is just that I don't. And as to taste, it may simply be my imagination or my aging taste buds, but it certainly doesn't seem that way. Food is prepared differently, and the ingredients take a different path from origin to table.

But what does all of that have to do with blindness? After all, that is what this book is about. Certainly blindness and blind people are not treated today the way they were sixty years ago. The blind of that generation had almost no chance to get a job, and very little chance to get an education.

In my case, I was allowed to go to college, but I wasn't permitted to take the course of study I wanted. I attended elementary and high school at the Tennessee School for the Blind in Nashville, graduating in 1945. One day in the spring of my senior year, a state rehabilitation counselor came to the School to talk to me about what I wanted to do and be.

Ultimately he told me (with big words and gently, but with absolute finality) that I could either go to college and study law and pay for it myself, or I could go and prepare to be something else and be assisted by the state. Since I was a teen-ager and didn't have any money, I went and prepared to be something else.

Of course, I now know that he was wrong. I am personally acquainted with at least a hundred successfully practicing blind lawyers, and most of them are not noticeably more competent than I am. But I would not want to create the wrong impression. This man was not trying to do me harm. Quite the contrary. He truly believed that what he was doing was in my best interest. He was trying to help me. He was acting in the spirit of the times and doing the best that he knew.

Today it wouldn't happen that way, for although there are still roadblocks and failures to understand, any blind person who is otherwise qualified can go to law school. And there are other opportunities, a whole range of options and possibilities for the blind that simply didn't exist in the 1930s.

Many things have made the difference, but principal among them is the National Federation of the Blind. Established in 1940 by a handful of blind men and women from seven states, the Federation has conducted a never-ending campaign to educate the public and stimulate the blind. I joined the organization in 1949, and it changed my life.

Today the Federation is the strongest and most constructive force in the affairs of the blind of this country, but its work is by no means finished. The job that still has to be done is not so much a matter of legislation or government assistance as of handling the interactions of daily life. We have come a long way in public acceptance, but sometimes the attitudes of sixty years ago are still with us.

Let me illustrate by what at first may seem to be trivial examples. Over fifty years ago, when I was a boy on the farm in Tennessee, I often found time heavy on my hands during the summer months when I was not in school. To relieve the tedium, I would sometimes ride with a truck driver, who collected milk from local farmers to take to a nearby cheese factory.

The days were hot, and when we could afford it, we sometimes bought a bottle of Coca Cola. (Incidentally, it cost five cents.) I didn't have much money, but now and again I had a little, and I wanted to pay my share. One day I said to the driver (a young fellow about twenty), "I'll buy a coke for each of us."

"Okay," he said, "stay here. I'll go in and get it."

"No," I said. "I'll go with you."

He was obviously uncomfortable and didn't want me to do it. Finally he said, "I can't do that. How would it look if people saw a blind person buying me a coke?"

I was a teen-ager, not yet accustomed to the ways of diplomacy. So I told him in blunt terms that I would either buy the Coca Cola publicly or I wouldn't buy it at all. After greed and pride had fought their battle, he decided not to have it, and we drove on--after which I was not welcome in the truck.

But that was more than fifty years ago. It couldn't happen today. Or could it? Well, let me tell you about an incident that occurred less than six months ago. My wife and I were entering a restaurant--an upscale, classy place with plenty of glitter and lots of manners.

It so fell out that another couple and we reached the door almost simultaneously. I happened to be positioned so that it was natural for me to open the door and hold it while the other couple entered, but the man was obviously ill at ease. He insisted that he hold the door and that my wife and I go first.

Since I already had my hand on the door and was holding it open and since I was not in the mood to be treated like a child or an inferior, I dug in my mental heals and stayed put. It was all done on both sides with great politeness and courtly manners, but it was done. As I continued to hold the door, the other couple preceded us into the restaurant. But the man was obviously uncomfortable, showing by his comments and demeanor that he felt it was inappropriate for a blind person to hold a door for him and behave like an equal.

Trivial? Not related to the daily lives and economic problems of the blind? Not a factor in determining whether blind people can hold jobs or make money? Don't you believe it! These incidents (the one fifty years ago and the one this year) typify and symbolize everything that we are working to achieve.

But again I must emphasize that we are not talking about people who are trying to cause us harm. We are talking about people who, almost without exception, wish us well and want to be of help. Our job is not one of force but of giving people facts.

And key to it all is the National Federation of the Blind--blind persons coming together in local, state, and national meetings to encourage each other and to inform the public. Sometimes we are tempted to believe that our progress is slow, but in reality it has been amazingly rapid. We have made more advances during the past sixty years than in all previously recorded history. And there are better days ahead.

It is true that the smells, sounds, touch, and taste of today are not what they were sixty years ago--but it is equally true that despite occasional nostalgia, we wouldn't want them to be. We wouldn't because today is better-- and not just in physical things but also in the patterns of opportunity and possibility. I say this despite all of the problems that face our country and our society. We who are blind look to the future with hope, and those who are sighted are helping us make that hope a reality.

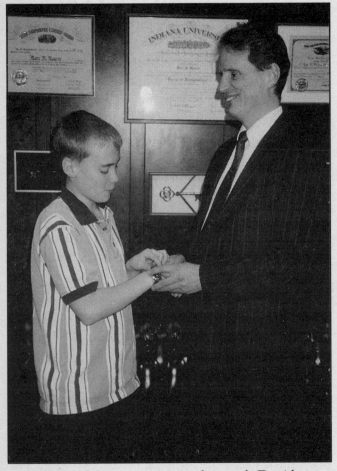

Marc Maurer examines the watch David purchased from a New York sidewalk vendor.

The City and the Fear

By Marc Maurer

A knowledge of the meaning of blindness is not automatic; it must be learned—or, in many cases, unlearned. When childhood fears are added to the mix, the combination can lead to frustration and anxiety.

Marc Maurer, President of the National Federation of the Blind, has two young children. Regular Kernel Book readers have followed the birth of his son David, their adventures in Cub Scouting, camping, cutting fire wood, and repairing the roof. Through all of it Marc has simply been David's father—who happens to be blind. But now David is approaching his teens. As he begins to absorb society's traditional attitudes about blindness, how will his father protect the relationship and keep it from deteriorating? In his heartwarming account of a family holiday trip, President Maurer explores this issue. Here is what he has to say:

In the Maurer household there are two adults and two children. My wife Patricia and I are both blind, but our children, David and Dianna, are not. David is thirteen and Dianna is ten. We are a family in the traditional sense—we go places together; perform family projects together; cook, clean, repair our home, and maintain our yard together; attend church together; and explore new horizons together.

We almost never discuss blindness. We don't forget it, but it is rarely a topic of conversation. Of course, in the planning for our activities, we remember that blindness is a factor. We do not own an automobile because none of us can drive it. So travel plans include hiring taxis, buying airplane or railroad tickets, renting automobiles and hiring drivers, calling upon friends and colleagues who have cars, taking buses, walking, using the subway, or some combination of these methods.

Then there is mowing the lawn and maintaining the yard. We do this as a family. My part of the job includes maintaining the lawnmower and other gardening equipment. We have a hedge, which runs along the front edge of our property. I keep this clipped, using a gasoline-powered hedge trimmer. If you touch the trimmer in the wrong place, it will trim your fingers along with the hedge— so I don't.

I also spend part of my time mowing the grass. However, this job is usually performed by David. My wife and daughter undertake to pick up the sticks and stray papers in the yard. The combination of effort gets the job done.

David and I mow the grass differently. He is sighted, and he watches what the lawnmower is doing. I am blind, so I use other techniques. I often mow under low-hanging trees and shrubs.

David finds this frustrating because he finds it difficult to see what he is doing. I can follow the shrub line or use the branches to tell me where I am and how much of the space has already been mowed. He uses one technique, and I use another. Working together, we keep the yard neat and tidy.

Inside the family there is no misunderstanding about who is in charge or how responsibilities are determined. The parents make decisions, and the children must follow direction. If the children misbehave, they are reprimanded or punished as circumstances warrant. They are given assignments and expected to carry them out, and they must seek permission to go visiting or engage in other activities away from home. This arrangement is stable and predictable.

Outside of our family this understanding is not always shared. From time to time we have encountered remonstrances from strangers. They tell my children that they must take care of their parents. They will stop my son or daughter on the street and tell them to be careful that I don't run into a telephone pole.

If I do run into a telephone pole, a thing which almost never happens, the children are sometimes chastised by strangers for their supposed neglect. My sighted children have been repeatedly told that they are responsible for their blind parents.

Sometime during the fall, Dianna asked me if we could go to New York. I was surprised. I have been to New York many times, and of course at one level of my mind I knew that she hadn't, but I simply wasn't thinking in those terms. "Would you like to go to New York?" I asked.

"Yes," she replied.
Can we?"

So, we planned
City.

Since I love m[y]
please her, we
immediately. Th[e]
When would w[e]
What would the[y]
it? I considered
Expenses durin[g]
been heavy, an[d]
budget could tak[e]
I am particularly
very much to gi[ve]
want if we can
aware that pos[...]
never kept.

There is always s[omething]
that interferes, or the
request to be made in
before the promise is c[arried]
these thoughts in mind,
should travel to New Y[ork]
Christmas. The Christmas dec[...]

rtainly like to go.

rip to New York

nce I like to
the trip
merous.
e do?
ford
ar.

ted to see
stay in the h
worried abou[t]
station and
way around
unrespons
the upco
he aske[d]
somebo
Dav[id]
he w
resp
wo[uld]

e the crowds would
holiday had passed.

still be in place, but David was not.
be a little sm... He asked if we could
Dian... ...to go with us. As the
...e nearer, he became less

He ...oud if there wouldn't be
...hment that would prevent
...o the trip would need to be
...old his mother and me that
...ything in New York that he
... He said that he would just
...otel and watch television. He
...t how we would get to the train
... what we would do to find our
... New York City. Finally, he became
...ve and irritable when we discussed
...ning trip. I wondered why, and when
...d once again if we could take
...dy with us, the answer became clear.

...id, my sighted son, was worried that
...ould be expected to serve as the
...onsible leader of our family—that he
...ld be called upon to know what to do

and where to go—that he would be required to make decisions and plan the trip. He felt that he was inadequate to meet the challenge and that he would be expected to shoulder responsibilities that were beyond him. He was worried that he might fail his parents and that his failure would cause distress or danger. Even if there were no danger, he thought the trip might be a failure because he would not know where we should go, therefore making the excursion to New York a disappointment, a disappointment that would be his fault.

As soon as I understood the problem, I knew what we must do. We would travel to New York and have a wonderful time. We would go together as a family, and we would do it alone—two blind parents—protecting, shepherding, guiding, and caring for our two sighted children. I decided not to tell David that I thought he might learn from this experience, and ultimately profit from it. Instead, I reminded him about all of the wonderful places there are to visit in New York. But it didn't seem to cheer him up at all.

On a Thursday morning, the day after Christmas, we boarded a train in Baltimore and headed for New York. I had hoped that the crowds would have diminished because we were traveling after Christmas. However, this was not the case.

The train was jam-packed. We had hoped to find four seats together, but no such luck. We settled for two. Mom, Dad, and David sat in the two seats; and Dianna sat on the suitcases at our feet. There was nowhere else to go and nowhere else to stow the luggage. You could say it was cozy, but you might also have called it cramped. Fortunately, the train ride from Baltimore to New York takes only a little over two hours, and the excitement of planning the next few days kept us occupied.

We had tickets for the Thursday evening performance of the Christmas Spectacular at Radio City Music Hall. We talked about visiting Rockefeller Center to see the tree and watch the ice skating. David wanted a chance to visit the toy store, F.A.O. Schwarz; and Dianna expressed a wish to shop at the Warner Brothers store because she especially likes Tweety Bird.

As the train halted in Pennsylvania Station

in New York City we stepped out into the cold air, and followed other passengers up the escalator. As we left the station, I welcomed the children to the sidewalks of New York— sidewalks as crowded as I ever remember them in the Big Apple. We found a taxi and loaded our bags into it. In a short time we reached the hotel, where we would stay for the next three days.

Our room was what you would expect in a decent New York hotel, but David (still mistrustful) wanted to know why it was so small and why it didn't have fancier amenities.

He had seen the Plaza in a movie, and he thought we ought to go there. I told him to quit griping and put his bag away so that we wouldn't stumble over it during our stay. I also told him to get ready for lunch, but he told me he wasn't hungry. I got the idea that he was more nervous than ever. But I was not prepared for his nervousness and irritability to become the controlling factors in the trip. I gave him his instructions: hungry or not, he was going to have lunch; so he had better get ready. I wondered whether the trip had been a mistake, but we were in the

Big Apple, and I intended to do all that I could to make our stay there enjoyable and memorable.

So the first order of business was lunch. In the hotel coffee shop Dianna and her brother both ordered chicken noodle soup, and they were warmed as much by the familiar food as by the steaming broth.

After lunch it was time to explore the city. We were planning to attend the early evening performance of the Christmas Spectacular at Radio City Music Hall, so on our way to the show, we decided to stop by Rockefeller Center (across the street from Radio City) to see the enormous Christmas tree and watch the ice skaters.

I asked the doorman at our hotel to give me directions to Rockefeller Center. We were on 47th Street, not far from Broadway. The doorman told me I should walk up Sixth Avenue to 49th and I would see it. He said we could get there in about ten minutes, so we started out.

The afternoon was chilly, and there were people everywhere. Street vendors offered us hot roasted nuts, hot dogs, soft pretzels, and hard goods such as sunglasses and electronic watches. But we were not yet acclimated to New York, so we kept on our way without stopping to bargain or buy. I was in the lead, walking with David, and Patricia followed with Dianna.

When we came to the corner of 49th and Sixth, we did not find Radio City, but somebody told us if we kept on for a block, we'd be there. And a block later, there it was. On 50th Street, we came to the skating rink. The crowds were enormous, and the line for admission to the rink was exceedingly long. We watched the skaters and admired the dazzling Christmas tree, decorated with hundreds of colored lights and a big white star at the top.

As the afternoon became evening, we joined the line for the Christmas Spectacular at Radio City Music Hall. The story of Christmas is timeless, but there are many ways to present it. Santa Claus told us that he couldn't do his work in one night all by himself, so he recruited helpers. In a few moments, there were sixty Santas on the stage. A moment later Dianna laughed in astonishment when animated Christmas trees danced in time to the music. Then, there was the story of the Christ child. My small daughter confided to me that she thought the camel (a real one), which was part of this segment of the performance, looked unhappy and confused.

David enjoyed the show, too, but he still seemed nervous. When we started back for the hotel, he thought we were going the wrong way. He imagined that we were getting more and more lost in this big strange city, but I told him we were all right, and sure enough we were soon in familiar territory.

When he saw the nut vendor outside our hotel, he obviously began to feel relaxed. He said to me that we had found the place, and without telling him that we had never lost it, I agreed.

The next day we started out for the toy stores, Warner Brothers and F.A.O. Schwarz. They are within a block of each other on Fifth Avenue, and across the street is the Plaza. This hotel, featured in the movie *Home Alone*, fascinated the children; and I promised to take them there for lunch. We did not merely eat;

we dined. The children asked for spaghetti, which did not appear on the menu, but the waiter said they would find some. The surroundings were elegant; the service was impeccable; and the bill, when it came, was as impressive as everything else.

Then, it was off to the Empire State Building. More than fourteen hundred feet in height, this tallest of New York buildings has an observation deck on the 102nd floor, from which we could see a cruise ship in the distance. A short walk from the Empire State Building is Macy's Department store, a central feature in the Christmas movie *Miracle on 34th Street*. On the way there, we passed more street vendors. Dianna bought a beret, and David purchased a Nike watch.

On Saturday morning we set off for the Statue of Liberty. This symbol of American freedom is over a hundred years old. We hired a taxi for the ride to the harbor, but we were puzzled about the place the ferry docked. I asked David if he saw the spot to board, but he did not. I told him I would ask some of the passersby where it was. He argued with me, telling me that they were ordinary tourists, not public officials. I said that they didn't need to be public officials to give us information and that they might know the answers to our questions. When I asked, they told us what we wanted to know. David was astonished and relieved to discover that this simple technique worked so well.

The method for finding your way is much alike both for the blind and the sighted. In an unfamiliar place, it may be necessary to ask for directions. If the directions are correct and complete, this solves the problem. If not, a request for more information may be made. This is how all of us learn how to get where we want to go.

On our ferry boat ride to the Statue of Liberty, we were at peace and enjoying the sightseeing as a family. David had stopped worrying that everything would go wrong.

He had been reminded, not in words but by example, that blindness does not prevent his parents from managing the family and protecting him and his sister. He came to recognize that he was not responsible for his parents but that the responsibility ran the other way. He felt good about this, and he relaxed.

In our walk around the base of the Statue of Liberty, a piece of history and the hope of the future came together. I could not help reflecting that the lessons learned by my children on the trip to New York are a small part of the process that will bring understanding and opportunity to all of humankind, including not only the blind but also the sighted.

Through the years, blindness has often been misunderstood, and that misunderstanding has prevented those of us who are blind from achieving our full potential. However, working together, we can change the negatives that have so frequently been associated with blindness. Sometimes it is done on the job, sometimes in a television appearance, and sometimes by what is written in a newspaper or a magazine. Sometimes it is done by a walk around the base of the Statue of Liberty on a holiday trip to New York.

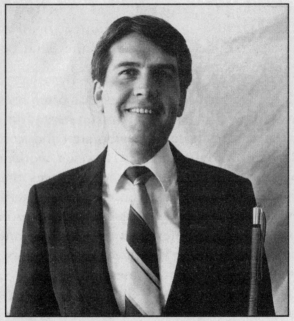

Bruce Gardner

YOU WILL HAVE TO MAKE OTHER ARRANGEMENTS

by Bruce A. Gardner

Bruce Gardner is President of the National Federation of the Blind of Arizona. By all of society's measuring sticks he is today in every way a success--a leader in his community and his church, a senior attorney with a major corporation, a member of the citizen's advisory council in his city, a scout troop official, a real estate owner. Just the kind of man you hope your daughter will find and marry. You do, that is, until you learn that he is also blind. Then what? Or what if the gentleman in question has not yet accomplished these things but offers only his high hopes for such a bright future? What do you tell your daughter and her young man? Do you tell them that they will have to make other arrangements?

These are the questions Bruce faced when he sought to marry Becca. Here is how he tells the story:

A girl I dated a time or two in college, after I began using my white cane, asked me to Sunday dinner and church afterward. As we left her apartment to walk to church, she turned to me and said, "Why don't you just leave your cane here. You won't need it at church because you will be with me the whole time." Although she was a nice young lady and I could tell that she quite liked me, I felt like saying, "Why don't I just leave YOU here." She had now confirmed what I had suspected--that she was embarrassed to be seen with my cane. She was not comfortable having others know that she was dating a blind man.

I decided to do both. I left the cane behind when we went to church for her sake. Then, for my sake, I left her behind when we got back.

Shortly thereafter I met Becca, and we hit it off immediately. She was very comfortable and at ease being seen in public, going places and doing things with a blind date. However, unlike so many others I had dated, Becca did not try to deny that my blindness could have an effect on our relationship. In fact soon after we started going together she told me that she did not want to get serious until she knew whether she could deal with my blindness. That was refreshing!

About a year earlier I had learned of the National Federation of the Blind, and I was finally beginning to deal with my blindness and come to know in my heart that it is respectable to be blind.

Becca was getting ready to leave on a two-week vacation, so I asked her to read a couple of articles while she was gone. I explained that the articles had been written by Kenneth Jernigan when he was President of the National Federation of the Blind and that they expressed how I felt about my blindness. She agreed to read them and when she returned from vacation, her ability to accept and deal with my blindness was no longer a concern to her. Within a few weeks Becca and I were engaged.

Becca's mother happened to be coming to Utah and planned to stop to see Becca, so we took that opportunity for me to meet Becca's mother and announce our engagement. She seemed happy for us, but she made a few troublesome comments like, "Don't worry Becca, I won't say a thing to your father."

A day or two later I met Becca on campus after finishing my shift as the supervisor of one of the breakfast crews at the dorm cafeteria. I asked Becca what her mother had meant. Becca said that her father was a little old-fashioned and that perhaps I should ask him for her hand in marriage. So I said, "I know where the pay phone is; I'll give him a call." Still I could tell there was something more to it. We were going to school in Provo, Utah, and Becca's parents lived in California. Even so, apparently her father had heard that she was dating a blind man.

When I made the call it was still early in the morning. Becca's father (a physician) was just getting into his car to go to his office, which was at the hospital. When he came to the phone I said, "Dr. Loeb, you do not know me, but my name is Bruce Gardner, and I have been dating your daughter Becca. I am asking your permission for her hand in marriage."

It would be an understatement to say that his response was less than I had hoped for. He said, "I do not give permission to marry my daughter to just anyone, and to me you are just anyone. You will have to make other arrangements." He then hung up the phone. I had the distinct impression that what he meant by "make other arrangements" was "go marry someone else."

When I hung up the phone, Becca asked me what had happened. In answer I said, "Get the phone book. I need to call the airlines; we are going to visit your parents." Those were the "other arrangements" I chose to make.

The earliest flight we could get was late the next day, which was a Friday. That gave us time to call Becca's mother to arrange for me to have an interview with Dr. Loeb at his office Saturday morning, and to relay to him, at his request, all the medical details I could provide about my blindness.

Of course I was scared. What was I to do? What could I say to this pediatric cardiologist that would alleviate his concerns about his daughter's marrying a blind man?

On Saturday morning when Becca and I arrived at her father's office, we learned that Becca was to have an interview first.

Only a few months earlier Becca had graduated from college and begun work as a registered nurse. Her father was concerned that Becca did not really love this blind man but only felt sorry for him and wanted to take care of him as she had done so many times before with stray or hurt animals and birds.

When it was my turn to be interviewed, I discussed with Dr. Loeb the medical aspects of my blindness, and he told me the results of his hasty research and conversations with the ophthalmologists he worked with at the hospital. We then discussed my plans to finish college and attend law school.

I also explained to Becca's father what my philosophy was regarding my blindness and asked him to read two articles written by Kenneth Jernigan, which would further explain how I felt. They were, of course, the same articles I had earlier shared with Becca: "Blindness--Handicap or Characteristic" and "Blindness: Of Visions and Vultures." Of course there was a lot of other NFB literature I could have given him, but these two articles summarized the issues well and had helped

Becca work through her concerns, so I used them again.

After my interview, Becca and I went to lunch with her parents and then accompanied them on their Saturday afternoon grocery shopping expedition, which was a weekly tradition. Although I was staying at their home in the guest room, nothing more was said either about my blindness or my engagement to Becca.

The next morning, which was Sunday, Becca and I were preparing to go to church. At the breakfast table Becca's mother turned to her father and said, "Becca and Bruce are going to church, and she wants to wear her engagement ring. So, have you made up your mind yet?"

With that her father turned to me, cleared his throat and said, "Did you have something you wanted to ask me?"

I just about fell off my chair. I muttered some lame apology for the awkward way I had asked the first time and then formally requested Dr. Loeb's permission to marry his daughter. He got a tear in his eye and a lump in his throat as he gave me his permission. He then excused himself and left for work at the hospital.

That was all there was to it. It was clear that he had read the articles I had given him and that he was impressed with the attitude I conveyed regarding my blindness.

I have since made good on my plans to finish college and law school, and for the past fourteen years I have been successfully practicing law. Becca and I now have six bright, healthy, happy children, three of whom are teen-agers. Since that interview with Becca's father, I have grown extremely close to her parents, and my blindness has not been an issue of concern for either Becca or her parents.

I am grateful to the National Federation of the Blind for helping me learn the truth about blindness and enabling me to share that truth with my wife and in-laws.

A WIFE'S STORY

by Theresa House

David and Theresa House and their four children live in San Diego, California. The House family is in many ways a traditional American family—David brings in the income and Theresa stays home with the children. And that's the way they both want it. It is also exactly the way Theresa knew it could be when she decided to marry David despite her family's grave misgivings. Here is what she has to say in this loving portrait of her family:

I am thirty years old, and I have been happily married for ten-and-a-half years. I have four wonderful children—three, five, seven, and nine. My husband David was diagnosed with juvenile macular degeneration at the age of five. He is now thirty-seven and has just a little remaining vision in each eye.

I knew my husband for several years before we actually began dating. His sister was my best friend in grade school, and as a teenager I was a member of the church youth group that Dave was in charge of. During the course of our friendship I was always impressed to see that Dave would never let

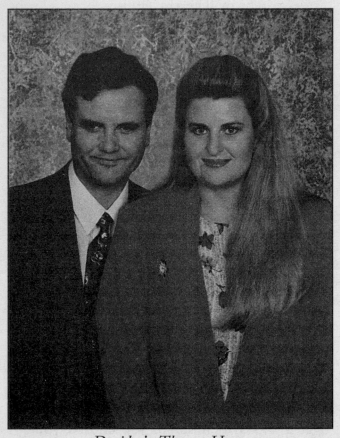

David & Theresa House

his blindness stop him from anything he undertook. A good example of this determination was the high school youth group of over a hundred teen-agers that he managed for nearly four years. Those years are very dear to me.

That group had the reputation of being one of the biggest and the best among the Catholic churches throughout San Diego. At the same time that Dave was our church's youth director he was attending San Diego State University.

After graduating from college, Dave made the decision to attend a residential training facility for blind adults in northern California. This was to learn Braille, cane travel, cooking, and independent living skills.

He believed that it was very important to learn the alternative techniques used by blind people before he lost his vision completely. Dave said that he was tired of faking and bluffing his way through awkward situations using his partial vision. He wanted to stop pretending that he could function normally in the sighted world by denying his blindness.

A year later Dave returned home to San Diego, well-equipped with the skills of blindness, full of confidence, and ready to hit the job market.

By coincidence we began dating the same month he was hired by Catholic Community Services. This was February, 1982. One of the fondest memories I have of the early days of our courtship was going out on dates riding double on my moped scooter. Dave did not drive, and I didn't own a car at the time. I was eighteen, and he was twenty-four. We still laugh today when we look back at that crazy and romantic time.

One of the more challenging aspects of our relationship was my family's prejudice about blindness. My parents did not approve of our courtship. They felt—and they still do, even though he has proved them wrong—that a man who is going blind does not have a bright future ahead of him. All this only convinced me that people's attitudes about blindness can be more of a problem than the actual loss of eyesight.

In 1983 we became engaged with plans for a June wedding in the following year. My family continued their resistance to my fiancé. When we got married in 1984, we were both working forty hours a week. I had a great paying job as a medical unit clerk in our local hospital. Dave had obtained his broker's license and was in the process of making a career change from social work to real estate.

A year later David, Jr., was born, and I cut my work schedule in half, to twenty hours a week. In 1987 our second son Christopher was born, and I reduced my work schedule to sixteen hours a week. Then in 1989 our third son Patrick was born. I decided to stop working completely to be a full-time mother and homemaker. I made this decision in the confidence that my blind husband was quite capable of being the sole breadwinner in our family.

My confidence was further reinforced in 1991, when we decided to have a fourth child. I was determined to fulfill my lifetime dream of having a daughter. My wish came true that year, and we named our beautiful little girl Veronica. For the past five-and-a-half years I have not worked outside the home because my husband has done such a great job of supporting us financially.

In our home, raising the children is truly a fifty-fifty partnership. After our youngest was born, Dave urged me to find a hobby so that I could take a well-deserved break from the kids in the evenings.

For three years I took martial arts, earning a second degree green belt in Tong So Do Karate. I am at the halfway mark of becoming a black belt, which I intend to accomplish. Also I am going to college at night, working to become certified as a floral designer. I plan to operate my own business out of my home doing floral arrangements for weddings.

None of this would be possible without the full support of my husband. Dave serves as an evening and weekend baby sitter whenever I have outside activities. My husband is no slouch when it comes to taking on his share of the chores and responsibilities at home.

Each day he helps me get the children ready for school by waking them up, feeding them breakfast, and preparing their baths. This allows me enough time for exercise each morning. I enjoy jogging. While Dave is getting ready for work, I make the lunches, help the children dress, and take them to school.

In the evenings after work, Dave assists me in getting the kids through their homework. While I am preparing dinner, he unloads the dishwasher and sets the table. After supper he clears the table, takes out the trash, and feeds the dog. In the meantime I am doing the dishes. Together we tuck the children into bed and then do paperwork, like paying bills and going through the mail.

My husband has found that keeping household items organized and orderly cuts down drastically on the frustration that can accompany vision loss. He has certainly proven this true by taking charge of the laundry for our family of six. Dave has used his Braille label maker on the washing machine and does a great job of keeping the clothes clean and neatly sorted. My job is to fold and put them away.

David makes blindness his responsibility and not an undue hardship on the family. For example, at home he has the choice of using his cane or possibly tripping over toys, shoes, or anything else inadvertently left on the floor. (We encourage our children to pick up after themselves, but in reality this does not always happen.)

Since I am the only driver in our family, I have been unanimously elected the family chauffeur. Dave himself makes it a point not to rely on me as his only mode of transportation. He makes his own arrangements to get to and from work, and he uses public transportation whenever necessary. He also enjoys walking places to stay in shape.

Dave no longer uses large print for reading because it is too much of a strain and too time-consuming. He says that, by learning Braille, he has kept himself from becoming illiterate. There are countless examples of how Dave uses Braille in his daily life.

I have already mentioned the Braille label maker, which he uses both at home and at work. My husband orders stories, called Twin Vision® books, which have both Braille and print as well as the illustrations. He really appreciates having the ability to read these books to our younger children. To help our older son, Dave orders a book in Braille that we can also find in the public library in print. This allows my son to practice reading aloud while my husband follows along in Braille, correcting him whenever necessary.

One favorite family outing is trips to the Price Club. My husband always brings an itemized grocery list in Braille to prevent us from spending too much money. Dave also receives the Sunday mass readings in Braille, which he takes to church each week.

He is a voracious reader, and between Braille and cassette recordings he manages to read a weekly newspaper, three monthly magazines, and a couple of books a month. I firmly believe that my husband is a living example of how blindness can be reduced to the level of a physical nuisance. In the event that total blindness comes, I know that he will be well prepared.

My husband is active in the National Federation of the Blind, which has over fifty thousand members across the United States. I can honestly say that the NFB has been instrumental in making my husband the self-confident, independent, capable individual he is today. The benefits and support Dave has derived from this organization have done wonders for his self-image and self-esteem. I would highly recommend the National Federation of the Blind to anyone who is struggling with losing eyesight.

A New Sheriff In Town
by Peggy Elliott

Have you ever felt you knew just about all there was to know about a particular subject only to find you still had a lot to learn? This is precisely what happened to Doug and Peggy Elliott (both long-time leaders in the National Federation of the Blind) when they brought a baby kitten who happened to be blind into their household. Here is how Peggy tells the story:

We have a new little kitten at our house. She's all black, but she had a tiny white star on her chest when she was born. It's grown in black now, but we still call her Sheriff.

Sheriff is four months old. Everything in her world is a toy to bat, chase, gnaw, or pounce upon. She is endlessly hungry, begs for everything, steals the two older cats' food, and sneaks on the table to cadge tidbits from us. Oh, and I should have mentioned, Sheriff is blind.

My husband Doug and I are both blind. We heard about Sheriff from a friend who took pity on a starving stray cat and soon

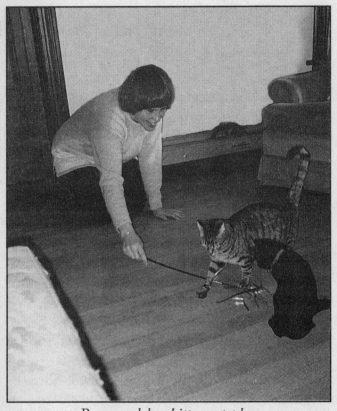

Peggy and her kittens at play.

learned the cat was a mom with two little kittens. When she was tiny, Sheriff put her head on the flank of one of her sisters to follow her to food and play. The little sister did not survive, and Sheriff had an incurable eye infection from birth that left her completely blind.

Our friend told us about his blind kitten, mentioning that he did not have any takers for this perfectly healthy, happy, bouncy kitten because she was blind. We knew what that could mean, and we offered to take Sheriff if no one else wanted her. We wouldn't give her up now to anybody.

We were worried about stairs, her finding the cat boxes, and interaction with the other cats whom we now call the Great Cats in comparison to little Sheriff. Here's how each of these worked.

At first we kept Sheriff in a room with a cardboard box across the door. This prevented her from getting out, but we and the Great Cats could get in. We were worried that, if we let Sheriff roam, she would fall down one of our two staircases, both of which have turns in them. We got a bell on a blue collar so that we could find Sheriff and avoid stepping on her. We would put the collar on only when we were taking her out of the room. She got so she purred when we put the collar on.

We tried to show her stairs, making her little feet look at the edges and risers. She didn't like the lessons. We made her go down, one stair at a time, to get the idea. She hated this. Then, one day about a week after we had Sheriff, we noticed that she was upstairs.

We had put her on the floor downstairs to play and gone about our business, keeping an ear on her movements, or so we thought. Suddenly, she was upstairs. It turned out that Sheriff knew all about stairs. There was a short flight in her original home in a garage, and she had used them from the time she was tiny. She still kind of galumps down the stairs, being a little too short from nose to tail to walk down yet. But she obviously will. She's taught us that. We tried to protect her, to ease her into our home a bit at a time. She wasn't having any of that.

We talked about this and decided that, even as long as we have both lived as blind people, we can still learn about the capabilities of the blind. In fact, both of us have had experiences where people think we can't do something and (from what they intend as kindness), prevent us from doing it. Stairs are one example.

We were recently in Washington D.C. visiting our Congressman, and we were heading out of the building to get a cab. As we approached the door, a Capitol guard prevented us from going any farther, telling us that she would "take us" to a door without stairs.

We had chosen this particular door because it got us where we were going. Had we been "taken" to any other door, stairs or not, it would have been a lot farther from our destination. We insisted; she relented, and we exited as planned, stepping down the stairs as agilely as sighted visitors. I couldn't help thinking of Sheriff and the help we had tried so hard to give her as I descended.

Regarding accidents, we simply haven't had any. We don't exactly know how she finds the cat boxes (we have two, one on each floor). We guess it is by using her sense of where she is as well as her nose. Early on, we worked very hard at being sure she was back in her room every two hours or so when she was a one-room kitten to be sure she would be near a box she knew.

Just like with the stairs, one day we noticed that a cat was scratching in the downstairs cat box, and each of us had a Great Cat on our laps. So much for thinking Sheriff couldn't find the cat box.

How about the other cats? GirlKitty is deeply suspicious of everyone but Doug whom she loves. Before Sheriff was even out of the carrying case in which she entered our house, GirlKitty was at the front door, glaring through the bars and hissing. In fact, we started calling her Miss Propane because she put her whole body into the effort, sounding like one of those propane tanks that cause lift in hot air balloons. She would even propane at Doug if he had been holding Sheriff, and she got a whiff of it.

In the early days, GirlKitty would punch Sheriff occasionally; you could hear Sheriff sort of go flying the other direction from the one she had been heading in. And once I think GirlKitty was actually holding her down and socking her—I was in the next room on the phone and, by the time I got in there, they were separated. But the thing we noticed most was that Sheriff never reacted to these expressions of disgust by GirlKitty. They were usually delivered right in Sheriff's face. But her body didn't move at all. We knew because the bell didn't tinkle.

We talked about this as well, relating it to our own experiences. Eye contact is crucial to cat communication, but it's very important to people as well.

GirlKitty seemed very puzzled that she was getting no reaction from her fierce glare and hiss. We have both known people who were very uncomfortable talking to us. It has often seemed to us that part of the discomfort comes from lack of eye contact and uncertainty on the sighted person's part that we can detect they are talking to us.

In Sheriff's case, of course, it just may be that Sheriff has better manners than GirlKitty. Anyway, she's found her own form of revenge. GirlKitty is very food-focused since she almost died as a baby from lack of nourishment. For a while, she said horrible things to Sheriff when the little kitten would try to join the Great Cats at the dry food dish. So Sheriff figured out that she could fit under the kitchen stool that happens to sit next to the cats' food station. GirlKitty can't.

So Sheriff gets under the stool and sticks her head out long enough to grab some food and then withdraws under the stool to eat. GirlKitty can't do a thing about it except stalk off in distaste. We didn't teach Sheriff about the stool. She figured it out for herself.

And then there's Bob, our large, mellow, kindly, clingy male. One day early on when Bob was eating, I put Sheriff on his back. Bob kept eating. Sheriff slid off on purpose. I put her back. Bob kept eating. This went on for a while because I was trying to teach Sheriff that one of the Great Cats was not a meanie. She learned.

When she finds Bob now, she jumps up on his shoulder or up his side in play. Bobby will sort of run and fight back appropriately, not knocking Sheriff across the room as he easily could but batting and taking evasive action as part of the game. They tussle like that. Then Sheriff loses physical contact and starts looking around with her paws for Bobby. (Doug calls her Scatters when she does this—running back and forth in very short spurts in a search pattern.)

If she doesn't find Bobby and he still wants to play, he will scrabble his back claws very fast on the linoleum or hardwood. Sheriff hears this and jumps. They start the cycle again.

Doug and I have laughed about this as well, having met people in our lives who are immediately comfortable with us, realizing that, although we respond to oral instead of visible cues, we are otherwise pretty much just ordinary people. Bobby got that idea right away with Sheriff. But he also tires of the kitten's endless playfulness. When this happens, he vaults over Sheriff and trots off.

Sheriff is still learning. When she came to us at six weeks old, she was too small to look at chairs with her paws and understand them. We would hold her in a chair and then put her down. She learned to climb up the upholstered recliner in her first room using claws, but she often misjudged and fell down before she learned.

She's now four months old and has a much longer wheel base from nose to tail. She has looked at the kitchen chairs with her paws, figured out how they are made, learned that they are comfortable, and now regularly hops into one or another. That is how she gets on the table. I now keep the chair next to mine pushed in all the way. Sheriff can get her head and upper arms up on the table but not the rest of her. So she sits there when I'm eating, for all the world like a little cat person except that she'd rather be on the table helping me with dinner.

And she applied her knowledge about kitchen chairs to all the other seating devices in our house. You never know now in which chair or sofa you will find her. We didn't teach her about chairs at all. By the time she learned, we had figured out that she did better learning on her own. We just get out of the way and let her explore. She does just that.

There are lots of other stories I'd love to tell: Like the fact that Sheriff gets in the middle of a wide open space like the kitchen floor and just plain dances—hopping and jumping and leaping to music only she can hear. Like the swisher toy we have—long strips of plastic attached to a rigid stick that you can shake in the air or tap on the ground, moving it around quickly for Sheriff to hear and attack, which she does with the same speed a sighted kitten would. Like the Great Cats hiding when the new bathroom was being put in while Sheriff hung around outside the door, listening and smelling and talking with the workers, as fascinated as the Great Cats were scared.

But I won't. Instead, I'll just say that Doug and I have been in the National Federation of the Blind for a long time and worked hard to learn that we can handle daily living tasks, jobs, home management just like our sighted associates. And we have both worked hard to spread that word to our fellow blind brothers and sisters as well as to our sighted friends. Even so, in the last three months, we've learned again the lesson of how easy it is to underestimate the capabilities of the blind. We were taught this lesson by a little black kitten we call Sheriff.

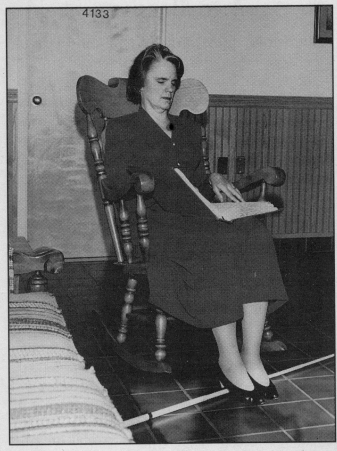

The simple pleasure of sitting quietly and reading a good book was long delayed for Barbara Pierce.

DICK AND JANE...
AND BARBARA

by Barbara Pierce

The story you are about to read is true. Unfortunately you could change the names, dates, times, and places, tell it over and over again, and it would still be true. We as blind people have enough real problems to deal with without having to continue to endure the needless illiteracy forced upon us by the failure to teach us Braille when we are children.

If you sense in my words something less than my usual good cheer and optimism, you are right; because the teaching of Braille to blind children is an area in which our schools have declined over the past decades, rather than improved. We in the National Federation of the Blind are working to reverse this trend, and we need your help to do it. In the following story Barbara Pierce lays out the problem. Here is what she has to say:

Can you remember the intoxication of learning to read? I can. When I began first grade, the Scott-Foresman primers about the adventures of Dick, Jane, and Sally were in use, and I still remember the picture of Dick standing on his head in a pile of leaves, feet kicking in the air, while one of his sisters intoned the page's text, "Look at Dick! Funny, funny Dick!"

Had I but known it, those early weeks of first grade were the high point of my reading career. We gathered around the teacher in reading groups to sound out the words and falter our way through each page. I was good at it. I understood the principles of picking out the sound of each letter and shoving them together rapidly enough to guess at the meaning. The result was that I was in the first reading group.

My success didn't last long. By second semester each page bore many more lines of print, and my mother was forced to work with me at home after school or before bed to help me keep up. For I was what they called a low-vision child.

I could see the print with only one eye, and I am certain that I was legally blind, though no one ever used that word in my hearing. Mother placed a little lamp close to the page so that I could see as well as possible, but the letters were still blurred, and I could never get the hang of reading an entire word at once.

By second grade I was in the second reading group, and by third grade I had slipped to the third group, despite the lamp now clipped to the side of my desk. I had to face the truth: I was dumb. I lay awake at night worrying about the increasing number of spelling workbook exercises left undone because my reading and writing were too slow to complete them in class.

I still maintained an unbroken string of perfect spelling tests because my parents drilled me on the spelling lists every week. The tests were nothing--but the workbook! I fantasized about what it would be like to go to bed at night and not stare open-eyed into the black prospect of mortification when the truth about me and my incomplete work eventually came to my parents' notice.

It happened at the close of the third marking period, and it came, as such things do, like a bolt from the blue. I had actually brought home what I thought was a good report card--all A's and B's--except for art, penmanship, and gym, in which I always got C's.

Everybody knew that I was terrible at those things because "Barbara's blind as a bat." But the dreaded unmasking of my shameful secret in the spelling workbook seemed to me to have remained hidden beneath an A for yet one more grading period. I handed my mother my report card and ran out to play.

But when my brother and I were called in for dinner (Dad was out of town at the time), I knew that something was wrong; Mother had been crying, and she did not sit down to dinner with us. She said that she had a headache.

It soon became apparent that I was the headache. My report card had betrayed me after all. In all that hard-to-read small print at the bottom the teacher had given me a U (unsatisfactory) in the puts-forth-best-effort category, where I was used to getting E's (excellent) or at least S's (satisfactory).

Mother went to school the next day and learned the horrible truth about me. I was astonished to learn afterward that the relief of having my shameful secret out in the open actually reduced my burden. True, I had to make up all the work I had been avoiding because the reading had become too difficult. Play time was much reduced, and I had to learn all over again how to go to sleep without worrying, but things were never again as bad.

In the following years we tried magnifying glasses for my good right eye, and the summer after fourth grade I had to be tutored in an effort to learn to read with high magnification. In September of fifth grade my new teacher called on me to read a paragraph in the geography book during the class lesson. I read like a second grader, and I was mortified.

The teacher never called on me again. By sixth grade I was hardly using the glasses at all. I was quick to learn as long as I didn't have to struggle to make sense of the print, and it was easier on everyone for the teacher to assign a rapid reader to work with me on in-class reading projects.

Finally, at the close of seventh grade, my parents faced the painful truth: if I were to have any hope of literacy, I would have to learn Braille. Print was no longer an option. I worked to learn Braille in a summer of weekly lessons taught by a woman who used Braille herself, though she admitted that she was not a good Braille reader.

She assured me that her husband could read Braille rapidly, but I never heard him or anyone else read Braille efficiently. People told me it was important to use my Braille and that practice would increase my speed. But by that point in my education I had already worked out alternative ways of getting my reading and writing done, and I was no longer eager to crawl down a page of text as we had done in early elementary school.

I practiced writing Braille with my slate and stylus because I knew that in college I would need a good way of taking notes in lectures, but I never made time to learn to read Braille properly.

Now that I am a member of the National Federation of the Blind, I know hundreds of people who read Braille easily and well. Some of them could not see print when they were beginning school, so Braille was the only option for them. But many more could make out print when they were learning to read, even though as adults they cannot see it.

They were lucky enough to be taught Braille along with print, and they simply and naturally learned to decide which method would be most useful for each reading task. As a result they now read Braille at several hundred words a minute.

I have never regretted learning to read print. Everyone should know the shapes of print letters, but I will always bitterly regret that I was not taught Braille as a small child.

Today I am struggling to gain the speed and accuracy in reading Braille that I should have had by the time I was ten. I have now been working at it for six years, and my reading speed has tripled, but I must face the fact that I will probably never read as well as a bright ten-year-old.

Setting aside the fact that the adult brain does not master new skills as rapidly as does a child's, I cannot bring myself to practice reading aloud to my long-suffering family. The time for taking advantage of such an opportunity is childhood, and I cannot inflict my stumbling reading on my husband.

If my mother could speak to parents who are facing the dilemma of whether or not to demand that their children learn Braille, she would urge them to decide in favor of Braille. No matter how clearly a youngster can see print at the moment, if the vision is fragile or problematic in any way, Braille will often become invaluable in the future, even if print too continues to be useful.

All young things need space to stretch and grow within their God-given abilities. Blind children must be given a chance.

THE OTHER SIDE OF THE COIN

by Ron Schmidt

Here is the other side of the coin. As you read this story, think about what Barbara Pierce wrote in the previous one, and think about what you might do to help us end the needless waste and pain. As is right and proper, we who are members of the National Federation of the Blind are taking the lead in doing for ourselves in solving this problem, but we can't do the job alone. Ron Schmidt is a husband, father, breadwinner, and Braille reader. Here is what he has to say:

I have been totally blind since age two. So luckily, no one tried to decide for me whether I should use limited vision for reading print. My mom read everything she could to me in my first six years of life, but it was never enough. Helping my dad run a busy dairy farm didn't give her a lot of free time to read to me, but I was eager to hear stories, as all kids are, and to learn as much as I could about the world I couldn't see. Reading other people's words (pictures of places and events and feelings) gave me a wonderful feeling of learning and understanding.

The most exciting event in my life as a child occurred when I went to a school, and my teacher said she would teach me to read and write Braille. Finally I would be able to read all I wanted, and about anything I wanted to know more about.

It was so much fun and so exciting that I never thought of it as schoolwork. By the third grade I had already gone through the Braille reading books our school had for children up to the sixth grade. I borrowed all the books I was interested in from the state library for the blind, and throughout the thirty-five years from then to now, I have been thankful every day that I learned Braille.

Through junior and senior high school and later in college I tried to get every course book I could put into Braille. It usually meant getting lists of books from teachers six months ahead of needing them. But all gladly tried their best to do it for me. It was always so much easier to understand and retain more of what I read by reading it myself with my fingers than to have it read to me by readers or by my use of recorded material.

Braille also allowed me to participate in reading aloud in class with my sighted classmates and to talk about what I felt with my family and friends. My roommates in college were always envious of my being able to read in bed late at night without any lights on, which they couldn't do without disturbing others who were trying to sleep.

As I write this, I am just turning forty-five years of age. For thirty-eight of that forty-five years I have relied upon the reading and writing of Braille for my happiness and success in school, college, career, and life overall. I read Braille books to my twin girls now and have since they were one year old, starting with the Twin Vision® books. I demonstrate Braille to their schoolmates and explain how it makes it possible to learn.

Getting my present job as a reservationist for the Homestead Resort depended (and, for that matter, still depends) on my being able to Braille pages of room and condo rates and other information, which changes regularly and which I must have at my fingertips to communicate to prospective vacationers when they call our office.

I use my Perkins Brailler, and my wife reads what I need while I dash it off at night and have it fresh at hand for the work the following morning. I doubt that I could have convinced my employer of my ability to handle the job efficiently enough to have been hired without the ability to use Braille.

There is nothing that makes a person feel more assured and independent than being able to write and read his or her own material--whether for work, education, or leisure. I urge anyone with children who have little or no eyesight to do all they can to get their youngsters to learn Braille. It is easier at a younger age, I believe, and can make a great difference in school and the rest of a child's life, just as much now as it did for me more than thirty years ago.

DELIVERING THE COFFEE

by Mary Ellen Gabias

Mary Ellen Gabias has held a variety of responsible jobs. She has worked for a state legislature and has been an administrator of a program which helps blind people find employment. Today she is a wife and mother with three small children. In her story, "Delivering The Coffee," she reminds us that it isn't always the great events of life that make the difference. Here is how she describes her own personal journey to confidence:

I was lucky. My parents always believed I could do great things. When I wrote my first composition in elementary school, my mother was very proud. She said that I could work hard and become a famous writer. She had it all planned. I would write "the Great American Novel" and make enough from it to support her and dad in their old age.

I began learning French in Grade 3. My parents imagined me working as an interpreter at the United Nations.

I became a political junkie in the seventh grade and began working on political campaigns in high school. My parents reminded me that I should not forget good ethics when I was elected to Congress. My parents definitely believed that I was capable of doing extraordinary things with my life.

It was the ordinary things that gave them trouble. I was expected to dust furniture, but my mother gave up on teaching me how to sweep floors when I couldn't get the hang of using a dustpan. I took my turn washing and drying dishes, but my sighted brothers were all expected to clear the table. It just seemed so much easier to do that job with sight.

I learned how to measure, pour, stir, and chop. I did not learn how to use the gas stove. In fact, my mother always thought I would have to marry a rich man, who could afford to hire a cook and housekeeper. Either that, or I should stay single and live at home.

My parents were quite progressive compared with some of the other adults I knew. They expected me to be responsible for myself and my actions. They pushed me to do more than I thought a blind person could do. They stood up to other adults who called them cruel for letting me play tag and roller skate. All in all, they were terrific.

But they had never heard of the National Federation of the Blind. They had very limited contact with blind adults who were earning a living and managing their own lives. The local agency for the blind had a very custodial approach. They organized picnics, but the people with the most sight served them food and cleaned up afterwards.

The totally blind people were taken to a bench and encouraged to sit there and wait to be served. My parents knew that I could do more than the agency thought a blind person could do, but they didn't know how much more.

I was a very typical adolescent. I felt ugly and awkward, and I was sure that every blemish on my nose made me a social pariah. With their usual patience and understanding, my parents reminded me that I wasn't the only kid who'd ever had a pimple. Blindness made me stand out more than any adolescent wants to stand out.

My parents helped me to understand that being different from everyone else could be tremendously positive, provided the differences were based on excellence and achievement. I came to believe that, if I were only good enough at everything I tried, people would forget I was blind and treat me like everyone else.

I became very active in the Junior Achievement program. High school students in Junior Achievement work with representatives of local companies to form their own small businesses. The businesses make a product or provide a service throughout the school year. If they are successful, they make a profit. If not, they go the way of many failed small businesses. Needless to say, the whole program is permeated with the spirit of friendly competition.

I was in Junior Achievement for three years. I worked hard and entered every competition for which I was eligible. In my senior year the other students in my company elected me executive vice president. I was very excited. This proved to me that people would forget I was blind if I was good enough at what I did.

Our company produced a radio show, which was aired on a local station. It was a lot of fun. Everyone had a turn being disc jockey for the week.

We sold radio advertising. We produced a company annual report. Our officers competed with the officers of 93 other companies for the title of "Officer of the Year". I won. Out of 94 executive vice presidents in northwestern Ohio, the judges chose me. What more proof did I need that blindness could be forgotten?

Then the wind was knocked out of my sails. I was told that I could not attend the National Junior Achievement Conference along with the other contest winners. They were afraid to be responsible for a blind person. They said I could go if I was willing to be the only student among the 2,000 who attended from around the country who came with their parents.

The conference organisers said they might let me eat with the other students, provided the food was not "too difficult." I could not stay with them on the college campus where the conference was being held. I would have to stay in a motel with my parents. I learned the hard way that others do not forget about blindness, particularly when they do not understand it.

I was not willing to attend the conference under such humiliating circumstances. My confidence was badly shaken. If being the best wasn't good enough, what could I do?

I first heard about the National Federation of the Blind when I was a university freshman. I read Federation literature with increasing excitement. Here were blind people succeeding despite obstacles thrown in their way.

They weren't asking anyone to forget that they were blind. They were not asking for special favors or to be taken care of by others. They were prepared to do their share of the work and to help take care of others in need.

As I met other members of the National Federation of the Blind, I began to understand what real self confidence means. I did not have to struggle to be perfect at everything I tried in order to feel acceptable to others. I needed to strive for excellence because doing my best was the right thing to do.

I met people who were doing things which I admired. Some were succeeding in careers I never dreamed possible for a blind person. Others were doing the ordinary work of everyday living with skill and grace.

Sometimes it is the small moments which make the largest impact. I was attending the Federation's National Convention during the summer when I graduated from college. The Presidential Suite was a place for convention delegates to gather, make friends, and conduct business with the President.

There was always a pot of coffee on hand to serve visitors. I dropped by the suite to say hello to friends. Someone asked for a cup of coffee and the person in charge said to me "Will you get that, Mary Ellen?"

That simple request threw me into a dither. I was an honors graduate of a large state university. I'd travelled by myself across the country. But, I had never before carried a steaming cup of coffee across a crowded room.

Yet someone had asked me to do just that. I was afraid I might not put the right amount of cream and sugar in the cup. I was afraid I might burn myself when I poured the coffee. I was afraid I might bump into someone and dump the whole cup on them.

But I was at the Convention of the National Federation of the Blind. This was not the place to use blindness as an excuse for failing to try. Besides, where else would I get more understanding and support if things didn't go well?

I delivered the cup of coffee. Nothing went wrong. In fact, I doubt if anyone else realized what a moment of truth this small act had been for me.

I was quite ready to heave a sigh of relief and rest on my laurels. Then three more people asked for coffee. Before long, I'd gotten over my nervousness. By the end of the afternoon, I felt quite experienced. I did drop a cup and realized the world did not come to an end. That was just an ordinary part of doing an ordinary job.

More than twenty years have gone by since that convention. I still enjoy writing and speaking French, though I've long since decided that the life of an author or interpreter is not the life for me. I'm still a political junkie, and I spent more than two years working for a state legislature.

Now I'm a wife and mother. I'm teaching my three-year-old son to pour his own apple juice. He's learning the ordinary skills of daily life from me. Now I'm the Mom who encourages my children to dream great dreams and work hard to achieve them. It's amazing how extraordinarily satisfying ordinary things can be.

ON WITH THE SHOW

by Patricia Maurer

Blind or sighted, all mothers tend to have one thing in common: They want their children to have better opportunities than they themselves had--no matter how good their own were. In "On With The Show," Patricia Maurer reminisces about her own childhood and shares her hopes for her daughter. Here is what she has to say:

Almost everyone dreams of doing something--something spectacular and out of the ordinary. Parents dream that their children will have opportunities to do things that they as children couldn't or didn't do. As a child I wished I could sing and play the piano and clarinet, but I didn't seem to have a talent toward singing or playing musical instruments.

My parents gave me the opportunity to take piano and clarinet lessons, and I sang in the school and church choirs. I could see only a little then and am nearly totally blind now. The teachers and my parents were not sure that I could get very far with my music, but everyone was willing to try.

I wore glasses, which helped me to see a little better. I used a magnifying glass clipped to my glasses to read print and musical scores. When reading music, I would read a line, looking very closely at the page. Then, I would memorize that line. Learning each piece was very slow and tedious. I did not seem to have any talent for learning to play these songs just by listening, although I did try playing by ear.

As you may know, there is such a thing as Braille music. To use it one must read it first and then memorize it, so that it may be played on the piano or on another instrument. I did not learn Braille as a child. I wish I had.

Recently, my daughter Dianna, who is sighted, began taking piano lessons. She practices each day and, her teacher says, reads music easily.

When it came time for her first recital, we arrived early and sat in the front row. Although I suppose Dianna was a little nervous, she did not appear so. When it was her turn to perform, she walked to the stage, seated herself comfortably at the piano,

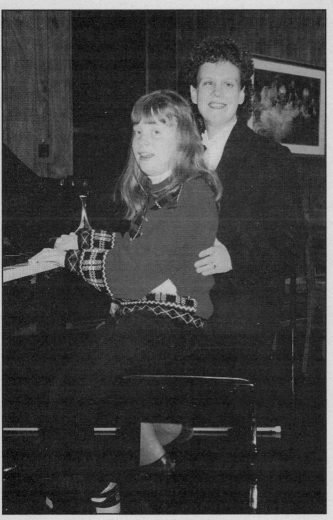

Dianna & Patricia Maurer

and played "On With The Show," the piece she and her teacher had chosen. How different the recital was for her than my recitals had been when I was a child!

I especially remember one time that I had worked and worked on a piece on the clarinet. Right before I was to go on stage, I could not remember my piece. If you have ever played the clarinet you know that becoming nervous definitely does not help your performance. To bite down hard on the mouthpiece produces a very squeaky sound. When I began to play there was only a series of squeaks. I was embarrassed and wished I were not there at all. My parents did their best to comfort me, but I am sure they were embarrassed, too.

I do not know if I would have done better if I had not been so nervous about going to the stage. Maybe it would have helped to have learned as a child how to travel with a cane and, more importantly, to learn that it is okay to be blind--that one does not have to pretend to be sighted. However, learning these things was not an option for me. There were not people around who could teach me. My parents did the best that they could, but they are the first to say how much better it would have been had they known about the National Federation of the Blind.

This incident, although embarrassing, has not damaged me for life. There are hundreds of children sighted or blind who are now adults and who can remember not doing so well at recitals--embarrassing themselves and their parents.

My daughter is not blind. She learns quickly. I know that today there are children who are blind who can competently walk to the piano or play the clarinet. They have had training and opportunities. There are still others who are afraid and need the chance to learn and succeed.

As I listened to my daughter play, I was so proud. Proud of her and proud of our family. We work together to see that she has a chance to learn. She will take that opportunity and do well with it. I also thought of my parents, and I thanked them for giving me the opportunities which they gave me.

Dianna is committed to doing well with the piano, and I am committed to doing my best for her.

So, "On With The Show." Who knows what the next recital will bring?

You can help us spread the word...

... about our Braille Readers Are Leaders contest for blind schoolchildren, a project which encourages blind children to achieve literacy through Braille.

... about our scholarships for deserving blind college students.

... about Job Opportunities for the Blind, a program that matches capable blind people with employers who need their skills.

... about where to turn for accurate information about blindness and the abilities of the blind.

Most importantly, you can help us by sharing what you've learned about blindness in these pages with your family and friends. If you know anyone who needs assistance with the problems of blindness, please write:

**Marc Maurer, President
National Federation of the Blind
1800 Johnson Street, Suite 300
Baltimore, Maryland 21230-4998**

Other Ways You Can Help the National Federation of the Blind

Write to us for tax-saving information on bequests and planned giving programs.

OR

Include the following language in your will:

"I give, devise, and bequeath unto National Federation of the Blind, 1800 Johnson Street, Suite 300, Baltimore, Maryland 21230, a District of Columbia non profit corporation , the sum of $\$_____$ (or "___percent of my net estate" or "The Following Stocks and bonds:_____") to be used for its worthy purposes on behalf of blind persons."

Your Contributions Are Tax Deductible